Fetal Alcohol Spectrum Disorders

Trying Differently
Rather Than Harder

SECOND EDITION

Diane Malbin, M.S.W.

Tectrice, Inc., Portland, Oregon
First edition published 1999. Second edition 2002
Revised 2011, 2016
Printed in the United States of America

Development of this booklet was provided by grants from the Children's Trust Fund of Oregon and the Office of Child Abuse and Neglect, Administration for Children and Families, U.S. Department of Health and Human Services. The State Office for Services to Children and Families, Oregon Department of Human Services, and FASCETS share ownership of this booklet. This edition is published by FASCETS, Inc.

To order this edition, contact FASCETS, Inc. at 503–621–1271
or www.FASCETS.org

Acknowledgements

Dedicated to Anya and Ariel, with love

This booklet was written to provide useful information, increase understanding of FASD, reduce frustration, and develop appropriate intervention and prevention strategies. It would not have been possible to write without the contributions of:

The many children, adolescents and adults with FASD who have taught us a language for understanding

Parents and professionals in the United States and Canada who have helped move information from ideas into action, through their insights, candor, creativity and determination

FASCETS staff, Judy Cropp, Connie Sirnio and Sunny Olsen-Kacalek

Sharon and Bud, for their vision and dedication

Diane Nowicki, for her invaluable guidance with this book

Wendy Temko, for her patience and persistence in editing the Second Edition

Hazelden, for permission to reproduce materials

Contents

Section four: Examples of Behavioral Characteristics and Effective Adaptations

Section Five: Comments, Questions and Resources

Fetal Alcohol Spectrum Disorders

Trying Differently Rather Than Harder

PREFACE

Many parents and professionals have been frustrated in their work with children and adolescents with Fetal Alcohol Spectrum Disorders (FASD). Good parenting and professional techniques that are successful with other children do not seem to "fit" for children with FASD. Too often, adults lack information about FASD and find themselves in cycles of increasing frustration, trying harder to change symptoms rather than trying differently.

A common misperception that "nothing works" surrounds people with FASD. While it is true that many people still struggle, we now have enough understanding of this condition to be able to support successful outcomes. For example, the University of Alaska recently graduated an artist with FASD who went on to earn her teaching credential and is now teaching art in a public school. In another city, during her recent high school graduation ceremonies, a young girl with FASD was described by her teacher as quiet, tenacious, determined, and an asset to her school community.

Anecdotal reports of people with FASD leading healthy lives are increasing in number. The following people are successful and they all have FASD:

- A drug and alcohol counselor and community organizer
- A teacher
- An internationally known musician
- An electrician
- A computer technician
- A husband and father
- A loving daughter
- A respected community leader

Stories of successful outcomes for people with FASD are still not widely known. These examples indicate there are effective approaches for living and working with children, adolescents and adults with FASD. Unfortunately, too many good parents and professionals still do not have information about why good standard techniques seem ineffective for children and adolescents with FASD, and what is more effective.

This book is about trying differently rather than trying harder. It introduces a framework for linking the idea of brain function with learning and other behaviors. This provides a way to think differently about the meaning of behaviors and develop different and more effective techniques.

Although the brain is complex, it does not require highly specialized training to be able to think differently about behaviors and develop effective strategies. The utility of the conceptual model introduced in these pages is not limited to alcohol-related neurological differences. It is a model which is believed to be appropriate for people with other kinds of organicity, including pre- and postnatal complications, traumatic brain injury, and some illnesses. This booklet simply supports the process of asking questions about brain function, linking this idea with presenting behaviors, and expanding parenting and professional options.

It is the purpose of this booklet to contribute to increasing understanding by providing useful, research-based information and examples of effective interventions. The goal is to expand parenting and professional repertoires, to prevent frustration, and to contribute to improved outcomes.

This booklet focuses on the effects of the drug alcohol instead of other drugs. Although there are about 50,000 environmental agents and other teratogens that may harm fetuses, the most thorough research has been on the long-term effects of alcohol. Illegal drugs, for example cocaine and heroin, were originally thought to be most damaging, but recent studies have found that the effects of alcohol are more long-lasting and damaging than other drugs studied so far.

Note: The field of fetal alcohol is relatively new, and changing terminology is common for new fields. The original term, Fetal Alcohol Syndrome (FAS), was expanded to include the term Fetal Alcohol Effects (FAE). In 1996, FAE was replaced by Alcohol-Related Neurodevelopmental Disorders (ARND). This term recently changed again to Fetal Alcohol Spectrum Disorders (FASD) and is used to encompass FAS, as well as the full spectrum of alcohol-related effects (SAMHSA, March 2003).

Section One

What is Fetal Alcohol Syndrome?

DIAGNOSIS

Fetal Alcohol Syndrome (FAS) is a medical diagnosis for a set of physical and cognitive (learning and other behavioral) symptoms of prenatal exposure to alcohol during pregnancy. The criteria for FAS are specific, and are at the extreme end of a continuum of observable effects. In order for a diagnosis of full FAS to be made, specific criteria must be met in three areas: 1) Small physical size, including head circumference, body weight and length, 2) Evidence of central nervous system involvement (brain differences affecting learning, activity levels, sensitivity and others), and 3) A collection of facial characteristics (small eye openings, thin upper lip, small jaw and others) . Please see page 79 for current diagnostic criteria.

There is a wide continuum of effects from prenatal alcohol exposure. People without full FAS are more difficult to identify since they may have few or no physical features. Now referred to as Fetal Alcohol Spectrum Disorders (FASD), this larger group is believed to be at greater risk for failure since they are not seen as having a disability. People with FASD may have significant brain differences, yet their behaviors may be the only symptoms of their disability. Because of this, FASD has been referred to as an "invisible physical handicapping condition" (Streissguth, 1996). Estimates of the number of people with FASD vary, although there is general agreement that this number is five to ten times that of people with FAS.

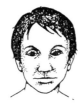

Child appears normal physically, but behaviors may indicate alcohol effects

Normal, given genetic background; may be exposed or have FASD

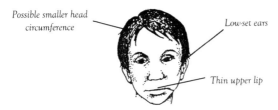

Possible smaller head circumference

Low-set ears

Thin upper lip

Has some "blunting" of facial features; may have partial FAS or FASD

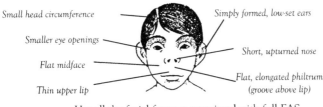

Small head circumference

Smaller eye openings

Flat midface

Thin upper lip

Simply formed, low-set ears

Short, upturned nose

Flat, elongated philtrum (groove above lip)

Has all the facial features associated with full FAS

FAS is at the extreme end of the continuum of observable effects. In the absence of visible changes, there may be changes in the brain. FASD is not necessarily the less severe form of FAS, but people with FASD are less likely to be identified as needing support. Please remember that any one or two of these characteristics may simply reflect genetic background rather than FAS or FASD. (Reprinted with permission from Hazleden Educational Materials.)

EFFECTS OF ALCOHOL ON THE DEVELOPING BRAIN

Research has consistently found the brain to be the organ most sensitive to the effects of prenatal exposure to alcohol and other drugs. The brain is growing and developing throughout gestation and is affected differently at different times. The timing of the exposure, peak alcohol/drug levels, genetics, nutrition, stress, age of the parent and other variables contribute to the wide range of effects. No two people with FASD are the same; different parents drinking similar amounts may have children with different effects. Not all alcoholics give birth to children with FAS, and some social drinkers do.

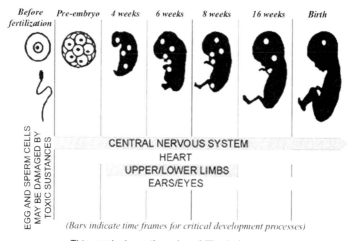

| Before fertilization | Pre-embryo | 4 weeks | 6 weeks | 8 weeks | 16 weeks | Birth |

EGG AND SPERM CELLS MAY BE DAMAGED BY TOXIC SUSTANCES

CENTRAL NERVOUS SYSTEM
HEART
UPPER/LOWER LIMBS
EARS/EYES

(Bars indicate time frames for critical development processes)

This graph shows the vulnerablility during pregnancy.
Note that the brain is susceptible throughout gestation and after birth.

The average IQ for full FAS is about 70. More importantly, the IQ range for full FAS is from 20–130. People with FASD who have none of the visible physical features of FAS and who have "average" IQs may still have significant differences in brain function. If alcohol is not consumed during the first trimester, during the time the fetus is forming, there will not be full FAS. However, drinking at any time during pregnancy (and during breast-feeding) may affect development. Stopping drinking at any time during pregnancy improves outcomes for both parent and child.

Alcohol kills cells. If large amounts are consumed, and enough brain cells are damaged, brains are actually smaller. The size of the brain dictates the size of the head, and a small head circumference is associated with the diagnosis of FAS. Even if microcephaly is not present, the brain may function differently. Recent diagnostic imaging studies of people with FASD show lesions and differences in the structure and function of the brain. Not all have observable changes, however. Other studies have also found changes in the neurochemistry in brains, with altered neurotransmitters and hormones.

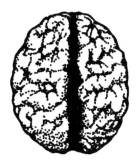 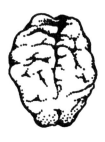

Apparently normal brain
at birth

Brain with FAS
at birth

PLEASE NOTE: The brains of most people with FASD are not visibly affected. This drawing is useful since it reinforces the idea that alcohol changes brains. Showing this illustration to people with FASD is not necessarily helpful, since it may be frightening, and may only send part of the message of how people learn differently. Remember that even with significant structural changes, many with FASD are able to compensate for these differences in creative ways with understanding, validation and support. (Reprinted with permission from Hazleden Educational Materials.)

IDENTIFICATION VS LABELING

Identification is distinct from labeling where "labeling" means limiting. Labels are liberally applied: people are labeled Talented and Gifted, Learning Disabled, Attention Deficit Disorder, Seriously Emotionally Disturbed, and others. A common concern about labeling people with FASD is that, unlike other conditions whose cause is unknown, FASD immediately implicates the parent(s): drinking caused this condition. It may be easier to diagnose ADD than FAS since this avoids naming the cause, but without identification of the issue, prevention efforts are compromised. Used supportively, identification provides a beginning, a way to develop a language for talking about FASD, and a way to develop effective supports for children and achieving prevention.

Identification of FASD is synonymous with recognizing changes in the structure and functioning of the brain and understanding what this means behaviorally. The brain is central to life, learning and other behaviors. Reframing the meaning of behaviors to include organic differences provides a shift for understanding people differently. Once the willful child is understood as having challenges, perception shifts from seeing the child as one who *won't* do something to one who possibly *can't*. This difference in understanding reduces frustration and increases successes. Such reframing is pivotal for creating a climate for developing effective and humane supports and preventing secondary defensive behaviors.

THE LINK BETWEEN BRAIN DIFFERENCES AND BEHAVIORS

Historically, the role of brain differences in understanding behaviors has not been systematically studied. Early research articles on minimal brain disorders were met with scorn from those who saw this as a way to "excuse" behaviors.

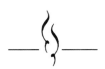

People with FASD live in a world that doesn't understand the link between brain differences and behaviors

Recent technological advances have increased our understanding of brain structure and function. Brain research has allowed us to expand our understanding of many behavioral symptoms of brain dysfunction. It now provides a way to approach thinking about behaviors very differently. Linking the role of the brain with behaviors is timely, appropriate and effective.

People with FASD have, by definition, differences in their brains. They have a physical disability. They may have no observable facial characteristics from prenatal alcohol exposure. Their only symptoms may be seen in primary and secondary behaviors. Thinking about behaviors as symptoms of a physical disability expands options for developing effective parenting and professional techniques.

Dr. Sterling Clarren tells the following story that captures what this means for caregivers and professionals. When visiting the library at the Center for Disease Control, he noticed that in each of the sections on physical handicapping conditions, the support literature focused on changing environments to meet the needs of those with physical challenges. Arriving at the section addressing behaviors, he was struck by how all the information in this section focused on changing behaviors.

What if behaviors are symptoms of a physical disability? Trying to change behavioral symptoms of this disability may be as effective as beating the blind child who "refuses" to read the blackboard. Providing environmental adaptations for people with behavioral symptoms of a physical disability is as appropriate and effective as for people with other, more obvious, physical symptoms.

People with physical handicaps are provided with environmental adaptations to help them reach their full potential. Depending on the need, wheelchairs, ramps, prostheses, guide dogs, Braille and assistive technology are provided. Laws have been passed to assure removal of architectural barriers, and prohibit educational and employment discrimination due to disability.

Children with FASD, whose *physical* disability includes brain differences, are often seen as having problem behaviors. They may get an "A" on Monday, an "F" on Wednesday. Without information about FASD, adults often see children with this behavior as lazy, unmotivated, or oppositional. If the children have FASD, the inconsistent performance may be normal for their disability. They are trying just as hard on "F" days as on "A" days.

Before their disability is understood, however, they are typically punished when symptoms of the disability appear.

The rest of this booklet explores the process of understanding neurobehavioral challenges and providing appropriate adaptations to support realization of the full developmental potential for people with this physical disability.

CONCEPTUAL FRAMEWORK FOR LINKING BRAIN DIFFERENCES WITH BEHAVIORS

Normal brain development is complex, with different parts of the brain and neurochemicals developing throughout pregnancy. At birth, hundreds of millions of neuronal pathways and connections are in place. This fundamental structure allows us to learn, store information, form links to generalize, abstract, weigh and evaluate, make decisions, organize, sequence, and predict. Even though there is greater awareness of different learning styles, and different kinds of intelligence (visual, auditory, kinesthetic, and others), basic assumptions about brain structure and function prevail. Learning theory is based on the assumption that brains all perform these functions. Entire institutions have been built on the principles of learning theory, which is fine for most people. However, this theory is limited in that it does not yet incorporate differences in brain structure that contributes to different kinds of learning and behaviors.

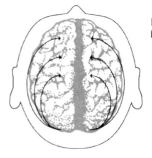

Learning theory is based on the belief that most brains function in a similar way:

- Rapid processing speed
- Store and retrieve information
- Think abstractly
- Generalize
- Predict
- Congruence between words, actions
- Understand and comprehend

Normal brain development is complex, orderly and sequential. Rich neural networks provide mechanisms for basic abilities: storing, remembering, integrating and retrieving information.

Alcohol is a very small molecule that passes freely into the placenta and fetus when consumed during pregnancy. It eliminates some cells, changes normal migration of cells, reduces the number of neuronal pathways, or connections between cells, alters neurochemistry, and reduces myelination of the axons, among others. In some cases, entire portions of the brain may be affected. Different structural and functional changes reflect which part of the brain was developing during the time of exposure. Memory, sensory responses, executive functioning and planning, processing speed, social and developmental growth and abstracting abilities are often affected.

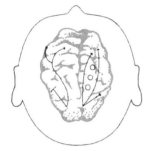

Neurological differences often appear as:

- Slower processing speed (thinking, hearing)
- Problems storing, retrieving information
- "Gaps", difficulty forming links, associations
- Difficulty generalizing
- Abstraction is difficult
- Difficulty seeing next steps, outcomes
- Disconnections: says one thing, does another
- Grasps pieces rather than concepts

With FASD there is often undergrowth, overgrowth, gaps and tangles. Because of fewer cells, brain structure and chemistry may be altered, affecting basic cognitive abilities and sensory responses.

Disorganization in the brain may mean that the brain has to work harder to achieve simple tasks. For one person, a task may be as tiring as going for a five-minute stroll. For another person with FASD that same task may require the same energy as performing a triathlon.

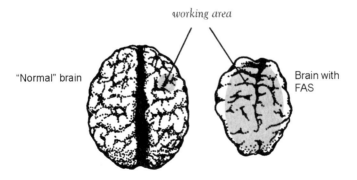

working area

"Normal" brain

Brain with FAS

PET scans are able to show which parts of the brain are working on a task. If two children are asked to perform the same task, a small part of the brain of the control subject might "light up" while nearly the entire brain of the child with FASD would light up. Alcohol causes disorganization in the brain, requiring greater effort to accomplish tasks. This often shows up in irritable behaviors.

Magnetic Resonating Imagery (MRI) studies have found some people with FAS to have visible differences in their brain structure. However, even those without differences in their MRIs may have significant learning and behavioral changes.

Lesions

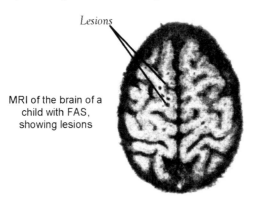

MRI of the brain of a child with FAS, showing lesions

Image courtesy of S. Clarren, MD.

FASD is not necessarily less severe than full FAS. Very few people with prenatal alcohol exposure may be diagnosed with the full syndrome due to the narrow diagnostic criteria. The brain is growing throughout gestation and after delivery. It is sensitive to the effects of alcohol/drugs throughout its development. There may be effects on the brain even when there are no external physical characteristics associated with FAS. These differences in structure and function may cause changes in behaviors.

Pathology drawings and simple diagrams hint at the impact of brain differences on people and their behaviors. They are useful cues for caregivers to remember to think "brain" when thinking about "behaviors."

It is fascinating to ask people with FASD to describe their brains:

- "If someone opened the top of my head and looked in, you know what they'd see? They'd see a whole bunch of black holes!"
- "My brain feels like Swiss cheese"
- "I'm the man with a mind like a steel sieve"
- "There's a wall in my brain. I know what's behind it but I can't always get over there."
- "It's like all the wiring is scrambled. Sometimes things just don't connect."
- "Inside my head it's like there are all these sheets of paper. Today they're all blank."
- "It's like there's a window in my brain and sometimes the window is open and sometimes it's closed."

None of these people, ranging in age from eight to thirty-five, had ever seen an MRI of brains with FASD. Yet their descriptions appear to capture the findings of lesions, or holes in the brain, neuronal disorganization, absence of the corpus callosum and other physical differences.

Section Two

Reframing Perceptions From "Won't" to "Can't"

Many books and articles have long lists of behaviors seen in people with FASD. Some of the behaviors make little sense when seen in a list (dysmaturity, difficulty forming links); others are frightening (anger, aggression). Recent research has attempted to unravel these lists of behaviors, creating new lists of primary and secondary characteristics (Streissguth). Primary characteristics are those behaviors believed to most clearly reflect underlying brain differences. Secondary behaviors are often defensive behaviors that are believed to develop over time when there is a poor fit between the person and his or her world, and when there is constant failure and frustration. These are often more challenging than primary behaviors, and are preventable.

PRIMARY BEHAVIORAL CHARACTERISTICS

Primary behaviors are behaviors that most clearly reflect differences in brain structure and function

- Dysmaturity, socially or developmentally younger than their chronological age
- Slower processing pace
- Impulsivity, distractibility
- Memory problems, inconsistent performance
- Strengths in some areas: art, music, interpersonal skills, computer, and others

- Difficulty generalizing, forming links and making associations
- Difficulty abstracting and predicting outcomes
- Over- and undersensitivity to stimuli

SECONDARY BEHAVIORAL CHARACTERISTICS

Secondary behaviors are those behaviors that are believed to develop over time when there is a chronic poor fit between the person and his or her environment. Like wearing tight new shoes whose constant rubbing causes blisters, a poor fit within the environment causes emotional pain. This contributes to defensive behaviors that reflect attempts to protect oneself from pain, and these behaviors are believed to be preventable. Defensive secondary behaviors may develop early, often becoming challenging patterns of behavior. Early identification, intervention and prevention are important.

- Fatigue, frustration
- Anxious, fearful
- Rigid, resistant, argumentative
- Overwhelmed, shut down (may demonstrate a flat affect and appear to not care)
- Poor self concept, feelings of failure and low self-esteem
- Self-aggrandizement, attempts to look good
- Isolated, few friends, picked on
- Acts out, aggression
- Family and/or school problems, suspension or expulsion
- Sexual problems (may be complicated by early sexual and emotional abuses)
- Truancy, run away, other forms of avoidance, trouble with the law
- Depression, self-destructive, suicidal (most serious and common among adolescents and adults)

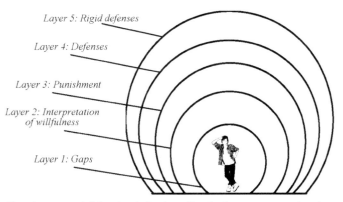

Layer 5: Rigid defenses

Layer 4: Defenses

Layer 3: Punishment

Layer 2: Interpretation
of willfulness

Layer 1: Gaps

Development of defensive behaviors: like the layers on an onion, layers of
interactions accumulate between the person with FASD and others.

Layer one: In this diagram, the first layer represents the request: "Johnny, please put your toys away, wash your hands and come to the table for lunch." Johnny does the series of requests on Monday, but not on Wednesday. He has "on" and "off" days due to his FASD, even though he is trying just as hard to comply on his off days.

Layer two: Without information, his mother's only interpretation of his behavior on Wednesday is that Johnny is being naughty, and deliberately playing. Because she thinks his behavior is willful, she becomes angry and punishes him since she wants to stop the behavior.

Layer three: When Johnny is punished for playing on Wednesday, he feels blindsided since he doesn't even remember what he was supposed to do. He gets angry and defensive, since he doesn't think her yelling is fair. As far as he knows, he didn't do anything wrong.

Layer four: The mother is doubly irritated by his anger since he seems "irresponsible." Now both child and parent are angry and frustrated (defenses are rarely unilateral, or one-sided), and this sets the stage for their greater reaction the next time something similar occurs (*Layer five*).

This is a common type of scenario, replayed in various settings, over time. It doesn't take long for both frustrated parent and child to be on guard, anticipating the next event. The defensive pattern of interaction often escalates, resulting in the use of increasingly punitive interventions. Eventually children are given diagnoses like Oppositional Defiant Disordered, Intermittent Explosive Rage Reaction, and others.

If behaviors are believed to be willful, intentional, or the result of emotional problems, interventions typically focus on changing the behaviors. If behaviors are understood as reflecting brain differences, interventions focus on changing environments in order to prevent frustration and provide support. (When people have both FASD and mental health problems, recognition of the primary neurological differences dictates the importance of treatment adaptations. This may include using art, poetry, drama, role-play, music, going into the home setting, and use of photographs to facilitate retrieval of information.)

The shift in thinking provided by understanding the difference between primary and secondary behaviors and the role of the brain in behaviors sets the stage for trying differently rather than harder. A common observation by parents and professionals is that the harder they try to change behaviors, the worse the behaviors become. When behaviors are used as cues, as symptoms of the disability, a different focus for interventions is identified.

DYSMATURITY, OR "ACTING LIKE A BABY": RETHINKING BEHAVIORS

Two hallmark characteristics of FASD that pose challenges to parents and other adults are social and emotional delays and memory problems, including processing speed. By themselves, these initially seem insignificant. The problem is that these characteristics are at odds with expectations for normal, or "appropriate" behaviors based on age. The world expects people to "act their (chronological) age." The normal behaviors of an earlier developmental level are seen as inappropriate, to be changed.

The following diagram shows a common developmental profile for an adolescent with FASD. In some ways, the person may be on time or even ahead of their years, yet in others they may be quite behind their peers. Imagine how problems could be avoided if expectations were adjusted to take into consideration this variability:

Timelines:

Chronological age ———————————— 18

Expressive language ————————————————— 23

Social maturity ——————— 12

Math skills ————— 8

Reading decoding ——————————— 14

Reading comprehension — 9

This diagram simply provides a visual for the kind of variability often seen in adolescents with FASD. A person may be 18 years old chronologically, and physically mature with strong expressive language, but developmentally, he or she may be much younger, socially and academically. Variability is normal.

CHRONOLOGICAL AGE AND DEVELOPMENTAL ABILITY COMPARISON

We expect children at age five to go to school, play well with others, take turns, and follow instructions. If the child is developmentally more like a two-year-old, it is helpful to "think younger," to adjust our expectations to reflect the developmental age.

We expect children at their chronological age to ...	But if the child is developmentally younger, they may ...
Chronological Age 5	Age 5 going on 2 developmentally
Go to school	Play at home, take naps
Follow three instructions	Follow one instruction, be shown
Sit still for 20 minutes	Be active, sit still 5–10 minutes
Play cooperatively, share	Engage in parallel play
Take turns	Always want their way
Chronological Age 10	Age 10 going on 6 developmentally
Listen and pay attention for an hour	Pay attention for about 10 minutes
Read and write fluently	Learn to write and read
Learn from worksheets	Learn by doing, experiencing
Structure their own recess	Need supervised and structured play
Get along and solve problems	Learn to problem solve
Have physical stamina, not tire easily	Become easily fatigued, overwhelmed
Chronological Age 18	Age 18 going on 10 developmentally
Be on the verge of independence	Need structure and guidance
Drive	Play with trucks
Graduate from high school	Still be dependent
Have a plan for their life	Be in the 'now', may not plan ahead
Have relationships, safe sexual behavior	Be immature, curious, impulsive
Act responsibly	Act responsibly for a younger age level

We assume abilities based on age. The gap for children with FASD is that they may be behaving responsibly, only doing so at a much younger developmental level. Seeing responsible six-year-old behavior in a sixteen-year-old looks like irresponsibility until the child's developmental level is considered. Before this is understood, these "inappropriate" immature behaviors often elicit fear, anger, accusations of irresponsibility, and attempts to change the behaviors. What if the child requires more time for more "responsible" behaviors to be learned? What if the timeline for achieving "older" behaviors simply needs to be extended?

Fights start when the expectations for "appropriate" behaviors do not include developmental abilities, and the level of expectation is too high for the child. We would not ask a seven-year-old to act like a sixteen-year-old, since that would be inappropriate. Yet we punish sixteen-year-olds with FASD for "acting" like seven-year-olds. What if the behaviors we see in the sixteen-year-old are appropriate for a younger child? What if he or she is being responsible, just at a younger developmental level?

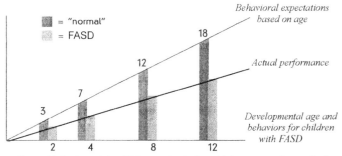

Burnout is "a deep state of fatigue or frustration which occurs as the result of a chronic discrepancy between levels of expectation and actual ability." (adapted from Freudenberger)

As children grow, expectations for appropriate behaviors increase with the age of the child. Behaviors seen as normal for a six-year-old are seen as increasingly inappropriate for an older child. The behaviors of a sixteen-year-old who "acts" like a nine-year-old are typically seen as irresponsible or inappropriate, and the child is more likely to be punished than supported. There is no time in a person's life when there is a greater gap between age and development than during adolescence. This gap causes distress for parents and a poor fit for sixteen-year-old children with FASD who are expected to function well with same-age peers.

Providing developmentally appropriate supports does not mean children are not expected to be accountable. It just means that the level of expectations for accountability is adapted to fit the developmental ability of the child, and that level is increased as the child matures, rather than ages. Behaviors seen as "responsible" are different for a six-year-old and a sixteen-year-old.

The long-term effect of the gap between expectation and developmental need is burnout. Children burn out and often act out, since by adolescence it may be safer emotionally to look bad rather than to look stupid, and adults living and working with them also burn out.

Burnout takes time to develop, and it occurs in spite of parents and professionals using good, standard techniques. The reason we get stuck trying harder to change children is partially explained by the following diagram:

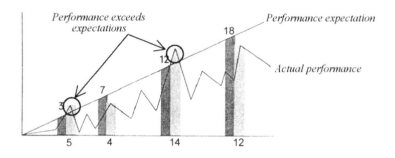

Having "on" days and "off" days, or inconsistent performance, is also common with people with FASD. Every once in a while, or in some ways, they meet or exceed our level of expectation. This provides random reinforcement for adults, which is the most powerful kind of reinforcement. It reinforces our belief that, "He can do it if only he tries harder. He's just not applying himself. With enough pressure, he'll do well all the time." Unfortunately, the child is trying just as hard on an "on" day as on an "off" day. It is more useful to recognize performance variability - this will reduce stress and anxiety. This suggests the importance of adaptability and flexibility for all adults who live and work with people who have FASD.

COLLECTING DIAGNOSES

It is not uncommon for clinicians to hear the following complaint from parents: "Our daughter has five diagnoses and is on thirteen different medications, and no one seems to know why. We're so frustrated! Our pediatrician is telling us to do one thing, the psychiatrist is telling us to do another."

Underidentification of FASD is still common. However, children with FASD often collect different diagnoses over time. There seems to be a common progression reflected in these diagnoses, with the earlier ones capturing primary characteristics and the later diagnoses reflecting challenging secondary defensive behaviors. In infancy and early childhood, children may be diagnosed with Failure to Thrive, Speech and Language Delay, Developmental Delay, Reactive Attachment Disorder and others. Later, diagnoses often include Attention Deficit Disorder, Learning Disabled, Obsessive Compulsive Disorder, Conduct Disorder, Seriously Emotionally Disturbed, and Oppositional Defiant Disorder, to name a few.

None of the other diagnoses are necessarily wrong, since these diagnoses are made on the basis of presenting behaviors. If FASD is also present, these other diagnoses may be incomplete and inadequate for developing appropriate interventions. They may not capture the central issue of brain differences associated with FASD.

Behaviors diagnosed as part of emotional disturbance, as mental health issues, often lead to diagnoses and therapies based on the behavioral symptoms (Axis I, DSM IV). While some people with FASD do have mental health problems, different treatment methodology is often required. Also, if parents and therapists expect a child to be "just fine" after treatment, the child will still have primary symptoms of FASD. This simply dictates the importance of redefining "just fine," since this often looks different than expectations for "fine." If the goal of the intervention is to change the symptom, and if the symptom is neurologically based rather than emotionally based, expanding expectations for outcomes is more supportive.

The problem with multiple diagnoses is that parents and professionals often labor under the belief that maybe another diagnosis will be the "right one," and that with the right diagnosis and intervention the child will become "normal." This can instead lead to confusion, complex and inappropriate interventions, and frustration.

COMMON DIAGNOSES ASSOCIATED WITH CHILDREN WITH FASD

The following list is a selection of diagnoses commonly given to people with FASD. There is a high degree of overlap between the behaviors associated with these diagnoses and those of FASD. None of these is necessarily wrong, but the presence of neurological differences dictates a different approach for parents and clinicians. The point is to ask the "What if?" question. What if some behaviors indicate neurological differences?

Consider this simple equation: The greater the number of diagnoses collected by a person, the greater the likelihood that something central, like brain dysfunction, has been missed.

- Attention Deficit Disorder, with or without Hyperactivity
- Reactive Attachment Disorder
- Learning Disabled
- Speech and Language Delay
- Pervasive Developmental Delay
- Developmental Receptive Language Disorder
- Sensory Integration Dysfunction
- Conduct Disordered, Seriously Emotionally Disturbed
- Borderline Personality Disorder
- Antisocial Personality Disorder
- Autistic, Asperger's
- Children of Alcoholics, Adult Children of Alcoholics

Attention Deficit Disorder seems to be the most common diagnosis given to people with FASD. About 80% of all children with FASD may also be diagnosed with ADD/ADHD, and about 60% of those with ADD/ADHD also have learning disabilities, etiology unknown. It is interesting to note that Attention Deficit emerged out of the literature on Minimal Brain Dysfunction. In 1966, Clements wrote three papers on minimal brain dysfunction, and listed ninety-nine behavioral soft signs of neurological differences. The professional community reacted to the complexity of the list of behavioral characteristics, and also complained that different interventions were not suggested. However, the idea of brain differences could not be ignored. Researchers identified hyperactivity as the most common symptom of Minimal Brain Damage (MBD).

Hyperactivity rapidly evolved into the concept of Attention Deficit Disorder. Observable behavioral symptoms formed the basis for the diagnosis; the idea of the role of brain function was mostly lost and interventions focused on changing behavioral symptoms through medication and behavior modification. In many cases, diagnoses of ADD are accompanied by prescriptions for Ritalin and recommendations for behavior modification programs. Again, while this may be useful for some, it may not be appropriate for many with FASD and ADD (See next section for a discussion on traditional behavioral interventions).

Although there are different causes of ADD, prenatal exposure is one. In some cases, behaviors reflecting neurological differences may be effectively addressed through environmental modifications. These should be implemented before other interventions. (This author is not commenting on the complex issue of pharmacological interventions other than to say they may be appropriate for some, not for others. See: Coles, 1997)

A gradual change in understanding behaviors seems to be occurring. Twenty years ago Autism was believed to be caused by "cold, aloof, intellectual mothers." Now, it is recognized as being a neurologically-based condition. The behaviors are not the result of bad parenting, they are the result of differences in the brain. The same evolution in understanding is occurring for ADD and FASD and other conditions as well. Twenty years ago children born with Down's Syndrome were institutionalized as unteachable. Now, many are mainstreamed as understanding and improved techniques have evolved.

Identification of the role of the brain provides an organizing principle, pulling together and making sense of a wide range of behavioral symptoms. As one parent said, "My son had seven different diagnoses. None of them was wrong, but none of them made sense of all the different pieces. We got the diagnosis of Fetal Alcohol and all the puzzle pieces came together and made a complete picture that makes sense."

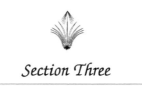

Section Three

Application

TRADITIONAL BEHAVIORAL INTERVENTIONS

Learning theory forms the basis for many parenting and professional strategies. This is fine, as far as the theory goes. Unfortunately, learning theory does not include recognition of brain differences. Learning theory assumes most brains perform basic cognitive functions of storing information, retrieving information, generalizing and abstracting. Unfortunately, people with FASD have difficulty in just these areas. Learning theory simply needs to be expanded to include different cognitive characteristics.

A closer look at the following learning theory-based techniques explores how they are all based on the same assumptions about brain function:

- Time out
- Extra work or chores
- Ignoring
- Shaming
- Star charts
- Contracts
- Grounding or other consequences
- Suspension
- Incarceration

In order for these techniques to be effective and result in changed behaviors, they all require specific cognitive and developmental abilities.

Problem: Johnny leaves his bike out in the rain. When his mother gets home four hours later, he is sent to his room for time out. The mother expects this punishment will result in a permanent change in Johnny's behavior, resulting in the bike always being put away in the future.

Learning theory assumes Johnny's brain can do the following:

1. Understand why he is being sent to his room, and remember riding his bike
2. Form associations between the bike, its location, and going to his room
3. Remember the unpleasantness of the time out tomorrow
4. Retrieve this information in the future
5. Generate different behaviors and predict different outcomes based on these different behaviors
6. Remember what to do with his bike the next day and forever in the future.

This is fine for some children. What if Johnny and others with FASD have difficulty in just these areas?

1. Linking words with actions, and understanding
2. Forming associations and linking the punishment with the action or behavior
3. Remembering, or retrieving information in the future, in different settings
4. Generating different outcomes
5. Abstracting and predicting future events
6. Generalizing information to new situations, in the future

Learning theory based techniques are not wrong. They just may not provide a good fit with the cognitive abilities of those with FASD.

Parenting differently rather than harder includes preventing problems instead of punishing them. This does not mean we allow bikes to be ruined, or otherwise tolerate challenging or problematic behaviors. It does suggest the importance of recognizing neurodevelopmental differences, and expanding our understanding of behaviors and of learning theory to include brain differences. Together, these help prevent problems and the need for punishment.

The point again is not that learning theory-based techniques never work. Rather, if the technique seems ineffective, it may be useful to explore whether or not the technique fits the person.

IDENTIFYING STRENGTHS AND TALENTS

A fifteen-year-old with FASD said, "I don't like having FAS, because I don't like not remembering things. But if I didn't have the FAS, maybe I wouldn't be such a good artist."

The young man with FASD who is now successfully employed building beautiful miniature landscapes for a nationally known architectural firm did not do well in math. As a boy, he had a train set and loved building miniature towns and landscapes. He continued to do this long after other boys his age put away their train sets. He turned his love and ability into a successful career. Is there coursework in high school for this? Could there be?

Primary strengths may erode if they are not recognized and encouraged. For example, if an athlete is prevented from playing sports because of low academic marks, his skill is devalued and the focus instead is on his deficits. This deficit model effectively gives the message that the person's strengths are not important, leaving the person defined by the deficit rather than by his or her strengths.

The following strengths are areas of interest and talents that often stand out in people with FASD:

- Music
- Singing, playing instruments, composing
- Art: fine arts or applied arts and crafts
- Spelling
- Reading
- Computers
- Mechanics
- Woodworking
- Skilled vocations: welding, electrician, mechanic
- Writing, poetry
- Others

These additional strengths may be built on to help support the learning process:

- Creative
- Often have strong long-term visual memory
- Friendly, loyal, loving
- Eager to please
- Determined
- Concrete, experiential, contextual learners
- Work well with their hands
- Learn by doing
- Learn by being shown rather than told
- Learn through relationship
- Learn through consistency, continuity, and relevance
- May be visual, kinesthetic, learn best when all modalities are involved

- Willing to work, though may require more time to finish, to achieve closure
- Perseverative

Remember the young man in the architectural firm? Although he played with trains into adolescence, his skill, strengths and interest were identified and encouraged. The behaviors of "immaturity" were not seen as problems, and he was able to grow at his own pace.

The goal is to provide adaptations that create a good fit between people and their environments, without limiting growth or enabling inappropriate behaviors to continue.

BUILDING ON STRENGTHS TO CREATE A GOOD FIT BETWEEN THOSE WITH FASD AND OTHER NEUROLOGICALLY-BASED BEHAVIORS

It has been said that parenting children with FASD is like trying to find your way around Denver using a roadmap of Portland. The map worked in one city, but not in the other. Using the wrong map is confusing, since some roads have the same name, but in Denver they lead to dead ends. Working with people with FASD is like developing a new map - not a better one, just a different one.

In parenting children with FASD or children with other neurologically-based behaviors, it seems like the harder we try to change behaviors, the worse they become. The shift in the definition of the source of the problem provides a different focus for interventions: from trying to change the child to changing elements in the environment. The paradox is that if we use behaviors as cues for recognizing an underlying neurological condition, and then modify environments to create a good fit, many challenging secondary behaviors are resolved or even prevented.

Environments are complex. Adaptations to accommodate the needs of people with many other physical disabilities are often fairly obvious: wheelchairs, ramps, removal of architectural barriers, Braille, prostheses, teaching sign language or providing hearing aids, and other adaptations serve to maximize developmental potential for people with other disabilities.

This simple idea provides a foundation for expanding our existing paradigm, or our way of understanding and addressing behaviors. It includes the idea of differences in brain function and helps guide exploration of brain differences and how these affect people in different situations. It provides an alternative explanatory theoretical basis for understanding symptoms of a physically-based condition, and from this, developing appropriate and effective supports and interventions.

Exploring the fit between people and environments starts with considering the role of the brain in behaviors and then recognizing neurologically-based differences. This then helps to identify strengths, sensitivities and other characteristics. Environments include both those elements received through the senses (sight, hearing, smell, touch, taste), and those that are more invisible (attitudes, perceptions, beliefs, values, timelines, assumptions, culture, and others).

Consider the following lists of characteristics in children and elements of environments:

Challenges and strengths for children with FASD	....And yet environments demand
Slow cognitive pace (10 seconds)	Rapid response
Dysmaturity, act younger than their age	Children to be grouped by age
Memory problems, often need reteaching	Remember after one lesson
Learn by doing	Abstract learning
Difficulty transitioning	Multiple transitions
Multisensory learners	One instructional style
Need more time	One timeline for everyone
Strengths: Art, music, work with hands	Value: academics

Many problems emerge when there is a difference between

adults' expectations of normal behavior and the actual abilities of children with FASD. The words "should," "knows better," "not acting his age," "not paying attention," "knew it yesterday, he should know it today" are often indicators of a gap between expectation and ability. The more a caring adult tries to change the child without recognizing brain-based behavioral differences, the more frustrated everyone often becomes. Accepting brain differences provides a way to accept developmental and cognitive differences, and on the basis of this understanding, to develop effective supports.

ELEMENTS OF ENVIRONMENTS: PHYSICAL SPACE

Physical environments are often stimulating and dynamic. People often adapt to environments by filtering out extraneous stimuli. Now consider the fit between everyday environments and the child with FASD: what if a child with FASD is unable to filter out stimuli? Imagine the chorus of competing sounds, smells, sights, and textures: fluorescent lights that flicker and buzz, competing noises from voices, radio, TV, intercoms, movement, decoration, outside activities, perfumes, physical contact, textures, decorations, and furniture, to name a few.

The challenge is to become conscious of all stimuli in an environment, and consider them for their potential impact on a person with FASD. Sometimes it is the 'little things' that make all the difference between comfort and agitation.

ELEMENTS IN ENVIRONMENTS: INVISIBLE, INTANGIBLE

Other elements in environments are often more difficult to identify since they are part of our paradigm, or operating systems. We are "in the middle" of our frame of reference, and it is often difficult to put words on these characteristics in environments. These include culture, nonverbal language, body language associated with emotions, effects of bias and prejudice, attitudes, values and beliefs.

Each of these elements represents bodies of history, experience, and norms contributing to the whole of the environment. Behaviors in children with FASD are often reacted to as being "at odds" with our expectations, values, beliefs and goals. These intangible elements are often more difficult to clarify and adapt.

GUIDELINES

The following guidelines are provided to support the process of exploration. The points are general and the questions are open-ended, to support identification of the wide variety of effects:

1. Consider the role of the brain, and ask the "What if?" question: What if behaviors reflect neurological differences?

2. Accept the person, depersonalize his or her behaviors, and establish a relationship

3. Stop fighting, step back

4. Observe patterns of behaviors, ask questions such as:

   - *What are the strengths of the person?*
   - *What is the developmental age of the person?*
   - *How does the person demonstrate hunger or fatigue?*

5. Consider the fit between the person and the environment. Think about physical sensitivity, developmental age, cognitive and auditory processing speed, memory inconsistencies, and symptoms of fatigue:

- *How does the person seem to experience the environment? Over- or under-sensitive to stimuli?*
- *What are the first cues for frustration and what are the circumstances?*
- *What is the information processing pace?*
- *Are there memory problems?*
- *Social problems? Friends or isolated?*
- *Are failures more a focus than successes?*
- *Does the person need structure, consistency? Has anything or anyone changed?*
- *What are the behaviors trying to communicate? Fatigue? Fear? Failure?*
- *What do you need?*

6. Invite the person into the discussion. Use concrete language such as, "Show me," "Is there a picture?" "What does it make you want to do?"

- *As appropriate, invite the person into the discussion.*
- *Identify "stuck points." Think of fatigue, consider time of day or week, and environment, e.g. is the instructional technique too abstract? Too fast-paced?*

PARADIGM SHIFTS AND PEOPLE WITH FASD

Parents and professionals report a significant shift in their perceptions about people with FASD once their disability is understood from a neurological perspective. As a result, feelings toward those with FASD also change, moving from frustration to understanding and acceptance. The following pre-post evaluation of participants in a course at the University of Wisconsin captures this shift. The column on the left contains descriptions of children with FASD prior to information on FASD; the column on the right contains descriptions six months later, after information on FASD was provided:

From seeing the child as....	To understanding the child....
Won't	To Can't
Annoying	Frustrated, challenged
Lazy, unmotivated	Tries hard, tired of failing
Lies	Confabulates, fills in the blanks
Fussy	Oversensitive
Acting younger, babied	Being younger
Trying to get attention	Needs contact, support
Inappropriate	Displays behaviors of younger child
Personal feelings from	To feelings of
Hopelessness	Hope
Fear	Understanding
Chaos, confusion	Organization, comprehension
Power struggles	Working with
Isolation	Networking, collaboration
Professional shifts from	To
Stopping behaviors	Preventing problems
Behavior modification	Modeling, using visual cues
Changing people	Changing environments

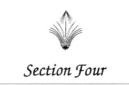

Examples of Behavioral Characteristics and Effective Adaptations

INTRODUCTION

The following examples were selected to illustrate some of the more common behavioral characteristics associated with FASD. In these stories, a situation is described followed by the standard interpretation of their meaning. Traditional interventions and their outcomes are described. This is followed by the introduction of information about the role of FASD in the presenting behaviors, adaptations based on recognizing both strengths and challenges, and different outcomes.

MEMORY PROBLEMS

Poor short term auditory memory, or forgets instructions

Example: A girl came home after school one day and dropped her coat on the floor under the coat rack in the foyer. She walked into the kitchen and said hi to her mother. Her mother asked her, "Did you put your coat away?" The girl said yes. The mother looked around the corner and saw the coat in its customary place on the floor and said, "Please hang your coat up." The girl said "Ok," left the kitchen and started walking through the living room to the foyer. Halfway across the living room she slowed down, paused, looked around, and started picking up the living room. After watching for a few moments, the mother came over to her and said, "Thank you very much for picking up the living room. Did you get your coat?" "Oh, right!" the girl said, and she went into the foyer and hung up her coat.

Intervention and outcome: Before learning about FASD, the mother would get frustrated when her daughter didn't follow through on the direction, and started doing something else. The girl knew she was supposed to do something, but forgot it was her coat, and so she started picking up instead. The mother also thought her daughter "knew what she meant" when she asked if her coat was put away, assuming she understood "put away" meant "hang up." When she saw it lying on the floor, she thought her daughter was lying or being lazy, and yelled at her. The daughter would then shut down and become angry.

Different intervention: After the mother learned about her daughter's poor short term auditory memory, that three feet away from her mother she would forget the original goal, the mother became less frustrated. She also realized her daughter was very concrete and specific, and that it was helpful to be very specific about how the coat was put away. This better understanding prevented frustration.

May need reteaching

Example: A parent of a ten-year-old boy was frustrated by having to teach him the same thing many times before he learned it.

Intervention and outcome: When the boy failed to remember what to do, the mother yelled, he was punished, given consequences, or grounded. Both mother and son were frustrated, since the interventions did not result in improving his memory.

Different intervention: Once his mother understood that he needed more reteaching than she would have thought he normally should have as a ten-year-old, she relaxed. She said, "I used to think he should learn it after telling him three or four times. I would get angry when I had to teach the same thing fifteen or twenty times. I thought he was doing it on purpose, at me, and I took it personally. Now that I understand it takes more times, I can relax. He's not doing it at me. It doesn't matter if it takes 30 times." She builds on his strength as an experiential learner and accepts the need to teach him the same concept in different settings.

"Talk the talk but don't walk the walk"

This phrase is used to indicate a gap or disconnection between words and actions.

Example: The mother of a now internationally-known musician told the story about how this gifted son could never remember the rules of taking off his shoes and hanging up his coat when he came into the house. Or, he would remember when he came in the front door, but not the back door. She said, "It made no sense to us that this bright, talented child could not remember to do these simple things." She was frustrated. Years after he left home, he came back for a visit with his five-year-old son. As they walked onto the front porch, she opened the door and started to welcome them in. In telling the story, she said, "Before I could say a word of greeting, my son said to me, 'Wait, Mom.' And I watched in amazement as he turned to his son and explained to him, 'When you come in this house, this is what you do: you take off your shoes and hang up your coat.' I didn't know whether to laugh or cry. He was able to tell his own son the rule that he was not able to apply to himself!"

This is a classic example of the saying, "Talk the talk but can't walk the walk." The ability to echo back words and phrases creates the impression that they "get it," understand, or can do what they say. Unfortunately, people with FASD often have difficulty connecting words with action. There may be a physical "gap" between connections.

Intervention and outcome: These parents recognized their son's musical talent at an early age. Although he had difficulty in school, his music was never taken from him. His strength was supported and he is successful, although he may still need reminding about some things in his life.

Discussion: If a person is able to say the rule but not follow through, check for comprehension and for the ability to apply what is said to what is done. Try saying "show me" rather than "tell me."

Difficulty forming links, difficulty generalizing

Example: A mother was teaching her seven-year-old son to walk safely to school. There was one busy street they had to cross on the way to school, so she taught him to stop at the corner and look both ways before crossing the street.

Intervention and outcome: The first few days, she took the lead and spoke the mantra: "Stop at the corner. Look both ways. If there are no cars, walk across the street." Then one day she asked her son if he'd like to lead the way, and he did. They came to the busy corner and he did the drill perfectly. Believing that he "got it" about safe street crossing, the next day he led again. But this day, they walked a different route to school, coming to a different corner for crossing the busy street. This time when he got to the corner, he walked straight into the street. Astonished, his mother pulled him back and asked him, "Don't you remember you have to stop at the corner?" His response was, "Yes. But you told me it was that corner, not this one."

Different intervention: This parent assumed when her son was able to demonstrate the appropriate safe behavior at one corner that he would "automatically" be able to do the same behavior at a different, though similar, corner. She learned that his difficulty generalizing meant she needed to check his understanding at different places, to not assume he "got it." He learned the piece, not the concept. She learned to check for comprehension, and was prepared to reteach him.

Discussion: "Don't ride your bike in the street" to a parent means ALL streets. The literal child with FASD will obey, and not ride in the street the parent was standing in front of when the rule was spoken, but may ride in another street. Failure to generalize dictates the need for reteaching until the principle is understood. It just takes more time, and usually more repetitions.

PROCESSING SPEED

Slow cognitive pace, need for more time to think, or "Ten second people in a one second world"

Example: A mother was frustrated by her son who said, "I don't know" to everything she asked. One day she said to her son, "Tell me the reason you say 'I don't know' so often." He said, "Because, Mom, you don't get as mad at me when I say 'I don't know' as you do when I don't say anything."

Intervention and Outcome: A rapid response time is valued in many settings - at home, school and community. We give timed tests, expect an instant answer to a question, and generally talk quickly. We often interpret a long response delay after a question is asked as being controlling behavior, which generates anger.

Different Intervention: People who need a little more time to find a response may learn to say "I don't know" in order to fill time and prevent punishment. This is a clever strategy for covering the need for more processing time. This mother invited her son into the discussion about her frustration, and learned about him from his insight.

Discussion: Provide time for processing. Depersonalize the behaviors, understanding that may take seconds rather than nanoseconds for a response. Time is a gift.

Slow auditory pace, or hearing more slowly

Example: An eighth grader was sent to the principal for a problem behavior in the classroom.

Intervention and outcome: The student sat in the principal's office in a chair across from his desk as he lectured her. He talked and talked, and soon she started giggling and trying to stifle her laughter. He became angrier and more frustrated as he kept talking. Finally, she could no longer contain herself and burst out laughing. He sent her home, and called her mother to tell her what had happened. As soon as the girl walked into the house, her mother said, "Mr. Phillips called and said you laughed at him when he was talking with you. What happened?" Her daughter responded by saying, "I went in and sat down and he started talking. He was going too fast and I didn't understand what he was saying, so I decided to watch his face. It got funnier and funnier."

Discussion: When people have slower processing speed, or "listen more slowly," it may take more time for the sound to connect with meaning. The experience is like hearing every third word of a conversation. Imagine.....able what.....to.....and.....don't,.....get.....it! What if you could only see or hear every few words of a sentence? Worse, what if you were also punished every time you didn't understand? When comprehending only a few words, the meaning is clearly lost.

—{)—

*Imagine…able
…what…to…and…
don't ,…get…it…!*

Children with FASD who have experienced this phenomenon since birth may have not received validation that this is normal for them. Without validation, they may be unable to develop a language for communicating this difference. They probably will not say, "Excuse me, I'm having a terrible time with my processing speed. Please slow down, use fewer words, or use visual cues to help me." Typically, what we see are behaviors that indicate the child is not "getting it." These may include shut down or distractibility. A first grader who does not comprehend may look out the window, climb under her desk, or get up and sharpen his pencil. What if the behaviors are cues for recognizing a need and providing support?

The harder we try to change behaviors, the worse they become. If we can recognize behaviors as cues for understanding brain differences and providing appropriate adaptations, then secondary behaviors may be prevented or resolved.

Technique: Think: "Ten-second children in a one-second world." When processing speed is recognized, appropriate adjustments become obvious. Provide adequate time, reduce the number or speed of words, and provide alternative cues. Also, think prevention by building on strengths. Understand the source of the child's original problem. Use fewer words, model behaviors, and use more concrete approaches for communicating.

DIFFICULTY GENERALIZING

Literal, concrete, and different logic

How often do we state a rule and assume the ability of the person to understand the principle rather than the specific? "He knew what I meant!" often suggests frustration when a specific directive is applied exactly as stated. "Don't hit Johnny on the shoulder," to an adult may mean, "Never hit Johnny or anyone else." However, a literal translation of the direction means Fred doesn't hit Johnny on the shoulder, he hits him on the arm instead. Imagine. He did exactly what was said to him, and may get angry if punished for hitting on the arm. Fred's behavior may initially look like conning, but it may instead be a literal translation of the direction.

Example: The teacher was mystified by a child with FASD in her first grade classroom who only learned to read a few words all year. Finally she talked with the girl and found out what her logic was: She could read the word "red" but not the word "car," since the "r" had already been used!

Example: Another teacher was talking with her class about numbers, and she mentioned number eight. A girl piped up and said, "That's the number that starts with S." The teacher insisted that when you spell it, it starts with E. They argued for a while until the girl came up to the blackboard and started writing the number 8, and the teacher could see what she meant.

Technique: Ask. There may be a different logic.

State-specific learning

Example: A girl studied for a test in her counselor's office. She went into the classroom, took the test and failed. She went back to the counselor's office, studied some more, again took the test in the classroom and again failed. Finally, she asked her teacher if she could take the test in the counselor's office and was given permission. She then aced the test. She may have been demonstrating the need to be in the same setting to be able to retrieve the information, or she may have needed fewer distractions. If her strength is that she is a contextual learner, needing to be in the same physical surroundings in order to remember information, this strength can be built on by making creative accommodations in the environment.

Example: Fred, a second grader, spelled the word "the" in class one day. The next day another child asked the teacher how to spell "the." The teacher turned to Fred and asked him to spell "the," and he went blank. Prompting him, she reminded him that it was the word he spelled yesterday. He thought and thought and then said, "Oh! Was that the word I spelled when Sally was sitting in front of me and Joe was sitting behind me and you were standing at the front of the class wearing a blue dress and I went t-h-e?" He seemed to need to recreate the visual setting in order to be able to retrieve the word.

Imagine how complicated life is when the visual context for learning must be recreated for retrieval.

Technique: Recognize the need for cues for memory. In many cases, use strengths to support retrieval of information, including visual cues (pictures, photographs), music, or others.

RIGID, INFLEXIBLE THOUGHT

Example: A family was seeing a counselor for information and support for their teen with FASD. One week, the mother said she was frustrated by the teen's constantly putting the silverware in the wrong drawer when it was her turn to do the dishes. "I tell her every time where they go, and she still puts them in the wrong place! She's doing it just to make me mad." There was a pause, and suddenly the younger sister said, "Mom! You rearranged the kitchen. I just remembered she's putting the silverware in the drawer where it used to go!"

Discussion: Inviting the child into the discussion may help adults learn that there is a logic to events, just a different kind of logic. This is often helpful for preventing frustration. Understanding the source of the frustration is central for preventing problems.

SPEECH AND LANGUAGE CHARACTERISTICS

There are many issues related to speech and language. The following characteristics are a few that have been associated with people with FASD:

- May have delays in developing speech and language; may have articulation problems
- May use incessant chatter, ask "nonsense" questions, use talking as "filler"
- May borrow words or stories heard from someone else or from TV, and may repeat as their own experience
- May "echo" or repeat words and phrases, but miss the meaning; may sound like they understand
- Expressive language is often stronger than their receptive language or comprehension
- May repeat instructions and rules accurately, but fail to follow through - the link between words and

actions may be missing (They "talk the talk, but don't walk the walk")

- May say the rule, state consequences for breaking the rule, then break the rule
- May confabulate - a function of brain damage where people "fill in the missing pieces." Sounds like lying.

Different technique: Step back from the words and think "brain function." Check for understanding and comprehension. Check for congruence between what they say and what they do. If there is a difference, make communication more concrete. (See discussion in other sections.)

PERSEVERATION; DIFFICULTY WITH TRANSITIONS

Once started on a task, there is a tendency for people with FASD to persevere, to "keep on keeping on," or to have trouble stopping until finished. When interrupted, frustration and anger may result.

Example: John, a second grader, was referred to a classroom for children with behavior problems due to his frequent tantrums in school.

Intervention and secondary behaviors: An evaluation of the circumstances surrounding his challenging behaviors revealed the following: John has FASD, has a slow processing pace, and is perseverative. When the teacher gave the class a page of arithmetic problems she instructed them to complete all the problems on the page. At the end of the allotted time, the children were told to put their work away so they could go on to the next task. John only completed half the problems and would refuse to stop. Even though she explained he could finish later, he insisted on finishing. Power struggles and frequent tantrums resulted. Attempts to stop his work were futile, since he was not done and besides, she told the class to finish all the problems. He was often interrupted in his activities due to his need for a longer time to finish tasks, and was chronically frustrated.

Different strategy: Once identified, prevention of the problem behaviors became obvious: adapt timelines, provide adequate time or reduce the number of problems so he may succeed in finishing. Use cues to support transition: adjust, anticipate, forewarn, use visual cues or adapt the schedule. In this case, the student's perseverative behaviors could be reframed as determination and a need to finish what he started.

Discussion: It may take longer for people with FASD to finish a task. Perseveration is often seen as controlling behavior, but it may instead reflect a need to achieve closure, to finish. There is often difficulty switching gears, moving from one task to another. At the turn of the century, Maria Montessori wrote of children's physically-based need to achieve closure. When interrupted before they have had time to finish an activity, the result is often irritability or frustration. Solution? Provide adequate time and adjust workload for successful completion in order to prevent frustration.

Difficulty with inferential learning

Much of what is learned is learned inferentially. Adults assume this and do not expect to have to teach "details." The expectation is that the person will learn many things without having to be taught. This may not be so for people with FASD. They may need to have information broken down and specifically taught to them.

Example: A girl learned to do arithmetic in school. She moved and went to a different school, and suddenly seemed to not understand arithmetic. Her mother took some of her work pages from the first school to the second school's teacher, and together they discovered the numeral "4" was written open on top at the first school and closed on top at the second one. The girl was unable to inferentially learn. All of a sudden, her four was gone. Other children would have seen the new symbol, tried it, and found it worked. This kind of flexibility was unavailable for the girl. She needed to specifically be retaught.

Easily upset by changes in the environment

Many people with FASD seem to rely on the location of people and objects in their external world for security. Any changes in the environment such as moving a bookshelf or rearranging a room, changes in the schedule or routine, or having different caregivers may be especially distressing and fear-provoking.

Example: One night after her son went to bed, a mother decided to rearrange the living room, and moved the stereo from one wall to another. In the morning, she was in the living room drinking coffee when her son got up and came into the room. She said, "He stopped dead in his tracks and got a look on his face. I asked him what was wrong and he said, 'Mom, if the stereo isn't over there, then where's the bathroom?'" The modest change in the environment caused him to feel disoriented and lost. Most people would look, adjust, and still know how to find the bathroom. It's hard to imagine what it would be like to have a brain that is so dependent on external visual cues in order for the person to not feel lost.

Technique: Recognize the importance of visual stability and the impact of change. Work with the person to accomplish change - in this case, rearranging the room. It is common to view children as being "controlling" in their reactions to unexpected changes in their environments. Reframe understanding to include the importance of predictability for security.

Difficulty predicting, seeing what comes next

Example: An often-told story that captures what it means to not be able to predict was told by a father in Nome, Alaska. One snowy day, he went to watch his daughter sledding. He stood on a corner at the bottom of a hill and could see his daughter preparing to sled down the hill. From where he was standing, he could also see a semi-truck approaching that was going to cross the sledding road.

Intervention and outcome: He waved to her to get her attention; she looked at him and he pointed to the approaching truck. She looked at the truck, looked back at him, smiled and waved, and zoomed down the hill. She passed underneath the truck as it went by, between the front and rear wheels, and came to a stop in the snow next to her father. As soon as he could speak he said, "Didn't you see that truck?!" She said, "Yes, but I didn't know it was going to go there." Again, it is hard to imagine what it would be like to have a brain which causes a person to literally be unable to see what is happening next.

Different intervention: Once recognized, the intervention becomes obvious: provide safety, prevent disaster, provide a "spotter," and teach hand signals for going or staying. These are appropriate and effective environmental adaptations. The problem occurred when the father assumed his daughter could predict the path of the truck and wait until it passed. He did not know she literally could not plan ahead.

Difficulty with time, math, understanding money

Example: A young man in a treatment center in Barrow, Alaska broke the 11:00 curfew every night; he would always come back at 11:15 or 11:30. The staff was planning to discharge him for breaking this rule. Just before this happened, he again returned after curfew and the staff on duty stopped him, pointed to the clock on the wall, and said, "Tell me what time it is!" He couldn't. No one had asked him if he could tell time on an analog clock.

Technique: Check for understanding and identify possible gaps in comprehension. Strategize with the person to develop strategies for success. This may include use of a beeper system, an inexpensive wristwatch with an alarm, a palm pilot for the computer literate, or another type of assistive technology to prevent failure.

Discussion: There are innumerable stories of children having increased behavior problems in school due to academic difficulties, especially with math and abstract instructional techniques. As children grow, there is greater urgency for them to not "get behind" in school, and this anxiety often leads to heroic efforts on the parts of children, parents, and teachers. Stories of students spending three hours a night on homework in the third grade are not uncommon. One family spent four hours a day, all summer long, with multiplication flash cards, so their fourth-grader would "succeed." The mother said, "I was frantic at the end of August because he still hadn't memorized the tables. We stayed up until 2:00 in the morning just before school started. He finally could regurgitate them to me, but he didn't have a clue what they meant. He couldn't use them."

HUNGER AND THE INABILITY TO LINK PHYSICAL CUES WITH NEED

Examples:

- A third-grade girl walks through the classroom knocking things off peoples' desks.
- A three-year-old has "out of the blue" tantrums and is inconsolable.
- A fifth-grade boy is on task in the morning, and has behavior problems in the afternoon.
- Day treatment staff comment that a child has "four-hour tantrums."
- Parents at a conference in Idaho complain about random tantrums.

Intervention and outcomes: All children were initially seen as inappropriate, aggressive, controlling, and were given consequences for their behaviors. The behaviors did not stop.

Different intervention: A closer look at the patterns of behaviors clarified patterns that had not initially been recognized.

For example, the parents in Idaho made the connection that the seemingly random tantrums were not random after all; they occurred just after their son attended "Brain Gym." He was physically (cognitively) exhausted. In other cases, challenging behaviors were found to be a symptom of irritability from hunger and/or fatigue. The attempts to change the behaviors were ineffective since they did not explore the cause of the behavior. All three children were provided with snacks and rest, and the problem behaviors were resolved.

OVERSENSITIVE TO SENSORY STIMULI

Example: A grade-school girl was able to sit still and pay attention in class until about 10:00 every morning. After then, she would be distracted, she would fidget, and not be "on task." Her teacher thought the girl could pay attention if she tried, so the teacher tried different approaches to help her sit still, but nothing seemed to work. Both the teacher and the child were frustrated.

Intervention and outcome: In this case, the inattentive behavior was the focus of the interventions. Initially, the teacher tried lecturing, putting her name on the board, taking away recess, and removing the child from the group. None of these interventions worked. The child had FASD, and this information was eventually provided to the teacher. She read that some children with FASD respond differently to their environments and observed the student's pattern of behavior over a few days. She became aware that this girl seemed to have a strong sense of smell, and seemed to smell things that others were unaware of. After she noticed this, she also became aware of the fact that at 10:00 the cooks in the cafeteria began preparing lunch. Since the classroom was next door to the cafeteria, those aromas were quite strong and distracting.

Different technique: After these observations, the intervention became clear and was elegant, simple and cheap. A useful technique for working with children with FASD involves asking children what is hard and what works. This teacher invited the girl into the problem-solving process by asking her to name her favorite fragrance. The girl said, "Lavender." The teacher bought an inexpensive sachet and gave it to the girl to put in her desk. The next day at 10:00, when the kitchen aromas wafted through the classroom, the girl brought out her sachet, smelled it, and the fragrance of the lavender overrode the aromas from the kitchen. She was able to stay on task.

Discussion: The point is that the behaviors were seen as a cue to think further about the cause of those behaviors, rather than targeting them as the thing to be changed. Recognizing their source opened the door for developing different and more effective options. The result was that the needs for both the teacher and the student were met.

It is important to ask and listen to peoples' descriptions of their experiences within their environments. People may have different kinds of sensitivities. Some may be bothered by the flickering, buzzing or brightness of lights. Others may have a strong response to being bumped or touched, and still others may have a strong reaction to loud noises. If people are feeling overwhelmed, they may seek out quiet places, for example, under desks, in closets, or out of the room.

Overwhelmed, overstimulated

A disorganized brain may have difficulty prioritizing and filtering stimuli. "Normal" environments may be overwhelming. Some children seem to have heightened sensitivity to sight, sound, touch, smell or taste:

Example: An adoptive parent told the story of driving in the car with her five-year-old son. She was cheerfully talking to him when he said, "Shut up!" Offended, she lectured him on manners and appropriate language. In retelling this event, she said a part of her brain neutrally observed his behavior as she lectured, noticing that as she talked he became increasingly agitated. Next time she talked when they were in the car, he again said, "Shut up!" This time she decided to be quiet and see what happened. He was quiet, settled down, and there was no scene. A few days later she was driving him to a friend's birthday party, and was instructing him on good manners. Again, he told her to be quiet, and she was. When they stopped at a red light, he started talking with her. She took the opportunity to comment on some party manners, and when the light turned green, both became quiet. "That's interesting," she thought. After a few more red lights and chat breaks, she decided to ask him what it was like for him when they were driving and she talked with him. She said, "He turned to me with his eyes wide and said, 'I see EVERYthing, Mom, I see EVERYthing!'"

Discussion: He was unable to tell her he was overwhelmed, and told her to shut up. She was offended and wanted to stop his behavior. However, when she stopped *her* behavior - the talking - observed his behavior, and then asked him what it was like for him, she learned he was trying to ask for less stimulation. Once that was understood, she could teach him more acceptable ways to make his request. At that point, both his needs for reduced input and her need for civility could be realized.

DYSMATURITY

Developmental considerations: The source for one of the most common frustrations for adults seems to be related to dysmaturity, or social and emotional lags. These are primary characteristics. The gap between chronological age and developmental age and related behaviors is one of the most important "gaps" for adults to understand about people with FASD. It is not unusual for a seven-year-old with FASD to "act" like a three-year-old, or a sixteen-year-old to act like a ten- or twelve-year-old. Unfortunately, parenting, educational, and treatment goals often focus on changing "immature" behaviors. That may be as ineffective as expecting a toddler to tie her shoes, or a six-year-old to do a research paper. Where there is a developmental gap, discomfort and fear arises.

This distress increases as children age. Behaviors seen as appropriate in a younger child are seen as increasingly inappropriate, or "immature" as the child ages.

Children are often age-grouped. If they are socially out of step or if they act younger than their peers, they may be left out or teased, and feel lonely and isolated. Some may mask their discomfort by clowning around, others may become defensive or angry, and others may withdraw. The secondary behaviors may be symptoms of discomfort.

Different technique: Recognize that the child is acting his or her developmental age. Extend timelines for maturation and achievement. Consider developmental age rather than chronological age. Time is a gift. "Think younger," or think, "stretch toddler," when working with children and adolescents.

Other examples of dysmaturity:

- May prefer to play with younger children, may play like younger children

- May be impulsive

- May be suggestible, peer-driven, or easily influenced by peers

- May require supervision appropriate for a younger child

- May not understand personal boundaries, may be "in your space," "in your face"

- May not grasp nuances, hints or oblique suggestions

- May be unaware of danger, i.e. may lack stranger anxiety

- May have an excessive need for touch, which is acceptable when 6, but not when 16

There seems to be a gradual catch-up potential for people with FASD, with the gap between chronological and developmental age narrowing after 25 or 30. There is no time when there is a greater gap between age and developmental level than during adolescence. Behaviors that were acceptable for a younger child are seen as increasingly "inappropriate" as the child grows up physically. It may initially feel uncomfortable to look at a seventeen-year-old and think "twelve." One mother referred to her son as a "stretch toddler" to remind her to think younger.

Again, the characteristics associated with FASD are not as great a problem as the poorness of fit between these characteristics in the child and his or her world. In terms of dysmaturity, most parenting books, schools and treatment settings focus on reaching behavioral goals that are "age-appropriate." These do not take into consideration developmental lags related to this physical disability. It is more effective to recognize and support the child developmentally, in order to create a good fit between the child and the world.

Comments, Questions and Resources

CONCLUDING THOUGHTS

People have basic needs: to matter, to be heard, and to make sense to themselves. When these basic needs of children and adults are unmet, frustration, confusion, and isolation often result. The purpose of this booklet has been to contribute to understanding the neurodevelopmental disorders of FASD; this understanding is expected to reduce confusion and to support development of a common language shared by people with FASD, parents and professionals to enhance communication about differences, alternative strengths and adaptations.

As a mother in Anchorage said, "After the conference on FAS I went home and told my son I learned what normal is. I said to him, 'Normal is just how you are.'" Normal may be different, not better or worse. And as an adolescent said about his FAS, "I don't like not remembering things. But if I didn't have FAS, maybe I wouldn't be such a good artist."

The goal of our work in the field of FASD is prevention, regardless of the point of intervention. The art is to communicate effective prevention messages without revictimizing the victims, or conveying messages of prejudice. People with FASD may be the innocent catalysts for expanding understanding of the role of the brain in behaviors. It is from this increased understanding that expanded options are generated to support people with this neurologically-based condition. This will then support changes on all levels, from the individual with FASD to the professional, and from programs to policies.

COMMONLY ASKED QUESTIONS

How long has FASD been recognized?

There have been references to the possible effects of drinking on fetal development for thousands of years. The first research confirming informal observations was conducted in 1899, over one hundred years ago. However, as recently as 1965, well-known authors asserted that "nothing could pass through the placental barrier," and that drinking during pregnancy was safe. Fetal Alcohol Syndrome was first identified in the United States in 1973. Since then, thousands of research studies have contributed to clarifying understanding of this complex condition.

How many people have FAS?

Most researchers agree that only about 1–3/1,000 people in the general population may be diagnosed with the full syndrome.

How many people are estimated to have FASD?

There are some estimates that between 15–35% of all pregnancies are "at risk" for some effects. About 80% of all people drink and about 90% do not plan their pregnancies. Normal social drinking often overlaps early pregnancy.

Do more Native Americans and poor people have children with FASD?

FASD occurs wherever people drink. Predictably, there are higher rates in communities where there is higher alcohol consumption. There is research suggesting the higher the educational level, the more alcohol is consumed. Prenatal care and nutrition also seem to play a role in the degree of damage associated with prenatal alcohol/drug use. There seems to be a differential in rates of diagnosis in different groups, however, with children of minority parents being diagnosed with FASD more often than children of white parents.

Do you have to be alcoholic to have a child with FASD?

No, and not all alcoholics who drink during pregnancy do.

How much alcohol does it take to cause problems?

Although this should be an easy question, it is complex. No safe lower threshold has been established. Social drinking has been linked with brain differences in children. One author said it is possible that one four-ounce glass of wine every ten days may be safe. There is research showing fraternal twins having different degrees of effects. Two women drinking similar amounts may have children affected differently.

I didn't know I was pregnant during the first two months and I know I drank a little. Do I have to worry?

There is no way to know with certainty. Since there are thousands of other possible environmental teratogens, any neurological changes may not be attributable to alcohol alone. Stopping drinking at any point during pregnancy improves outcomes for mothers and infants.

Does fathers' drinking affect pregnancy outcome?

There has been some research on the effects of fathers' drinking on pregnancy outcome, when mothers do not drink or use other drugs during pregnancy. Paternal use prior to conception does not cause full FAS. Research has linked fathers' use of alcohol with subtle neurological differences in their offspring: lower birth weight, higher rates of attentional problems (Attention Deficit Disorder), changes in activity levels (Hyperactivity), and other learning disabilities (e.g. Dyslexia).

If a person has FASD will their children also have FASD if they don't drink?

No. Fetal Alcohol Spectrum Disorders is the term used for the effects of alcohol on the fetus during pregnancy. However, this is really a sophisticated research question. It is asking whether or not the ovum of females with FASD have been affected prenatally, since girls are born with all their ovum. Although some research has found higher rates of birth defects in the grandchildren of alcoholics, even if their parents don't drink or use during pregnancy (Friedler), there is disagreement about this in the professional community.

How do I know for sure if my child has FAS or FASD if there is no prenatal history? Do I have to wait to do things differently if I don't have this history?

According to the Institute of Medicine, the diagnosis of FAS is specific and may be made in the absence of a maternal prenatal history. Diagnosis of FASD is much more complicated. Since there are many environmental teratogens that potentially cause neurological changes, it may not be possible to identify which are specifically the result of exposure to alcohol. Obtaining evaluations that include neurological and developmental components will help clarify learning strengths and challenges. Using the model of providing environmental adaptations to create a good fit is believed to be appropriate for all people, especially those with FASD.

I don't want my child to "get away" with bad behavior. How do I know what's FASD and what's on purpose?

Usually observing patterns of behaviors over time, without interpreting them either as willful or organically-based, will clarify their function. The goal of including the idea of brain function in understanding behaviors is to neither limit nor enable. The goal of the shift in perceptions is to be proactive, rather than reactive. Explore the idea of both primary behaviors and secondary defensive behaviors and think about unmet needs and characteristics in the environment to support the process of exploration.

When I treat my child like a younger child, I hear I'm babying her, that I'm overprotective.

One of the biggest challenges to parents is to use good parenting techniques that are at odds with community norms. Professionals typically share the same set of beliefs about the definition of "appropriate" (age-related) behaviors, and may not understand the importance of linking the child's developmental age into parenting techniques. This requires strength, determination, and willingness to educate others about FASD - family, friends and professionals.

I thought doctors, teachers, and other professionals would all have this information by now, yet it seems like I have to educate everyone I come in contact with about my son.

We like to think professionals have more information about important issues than we do, yet in this case there is often a role reversal. Parents often have more knowledge about FASD, since this information is not yet included in most professional curricula. This role reversal may cause some discomfort, both for parents and professionals. The value of teaching ourselves and sharing information, whether we are parents or professionals, is that ultimately the information will help not only the child, but also all who are involved.

I'm a teacher and just went to a conference on FASD. I can think of four children I've worked with who I now realize may have had FASD. I feel terrible now about how frustrated I was with them.

Grief and guilt about FASD is not limited to biological parents who learn about this condition and the effects of their drinking on their child. The depth of the grief seems to be as deep for foster and adoptive parents, family members, and many professionals, although the source is different. Most people feel terrible about how they treated the child prior to learning about FASD. It is crucial for us to be gentle with ourselves, and accept that we couldn't know what we didn't know. Find someone safe to talk with about the experiences and feelings.

I have thirty-four other children in my classroom. I can' change everything for one child

Rather than writing Individual Education Plans for all thirty-five students, it is more effective to write the IEP for the environment. The teacher in the story about the lavender sachet explained the student's need to her classmates, and the children understood and accepted the difference. She was able to communicate that "fair" is not "same." See other publications for examples of IEPs for environments.

Don't tell me behavior modification doesn't work. I can use behavior modification on amoebae in the lab.

Behavior modification is neither good nor bad, but it is useful to explore the assumptions on which its effectiveness is predicated. The expectations for behavioral changes at the level of operant conditioning of amoebae are considerably different than the expectations for behavioral changes in children. (See: Kohn, "Punished by Rewards")

Every year we seem to get the latest "pop" diagnosis, like a fad. How do we know FASD isn't just one more in a long line of hit topics?

How many people drink? Is it probable that drinking patterns will change dramatically in the next year or two? The conceptual framework introduced to support children with FASD incorporates the idea that brain differences may affect learning and other behaviors. This foundation is believed to support children with other neurologically based conditions, including traumatic brain injury, some serious illnesses, and others. It provides an alternative basis for thinking about behaviors, giving equal weight to the idea that the brain affects behaviors, and this concept appears to be timely and appropriate.

I just learned about FASD and find that I'm absolutely furious with the mothers who drank during pregnancy.

FASD is a hot topic, bringing up powerful emotions: anger, sadness, loss, shame, and others. The feelings are instructive, and are helpful in identifying our beliefs about others and ourselves. Many times the rage directed toward mothers is the result of beliefs that alcoholism is a moral issue, and that women, especially, who drink are choosing to harm their innocent child. Often the degree of the anger is related to how addictions have negatively impacted the person. The person who was physically or sexually abused by an alcoholic, who never witnessed recovery, may carry unresolved issues. Anger may reflect pain or frustration, and is part of a process. The question is how to direct the energy born of the anger - proactively or reactively. Proactive work seems to contribute to prevention more effectively than reactive, punitive approaches.

I'm not interested in diagnosing, just in getting more information to support a referral for a diagnosis. I don't know how to talk with the parents, even to get information. I'm worried they'll get mad, or walk out!

Can you think of one person that you know who has a problem with drinking or using other drugs? Have you been able to talk with that person directly about their drinking or using? Most people say yes to the first question, and no to the second. Discomfort related to talking about drinking has deep historical, gender, and cultural roots. It leads to most people not having a language for even talking about drinking. Discomfort may be normal; the challenge is to learn to develop a language and learn to talk.

As an Ob/Gyn, I find I am uncomfortable asking questions about drinking during pregnancy. I don't want to sound like I'm judging.

Although it is difficult to talk with both men and women about drinking, it is often more difficult to talk with women. One source of the discomfort also has a long history. In ancient Rome and Greece, women who were found drinking were severely punished. It was thought that a woman with wine on her breath was loose, promiscuous, a slut. Historically, women have been placed in the morally superior position to men, with images of purity, motherhood and nurturing surrounding their role. The image of the drinking whore is at direct odds with this image. The "stigma" associated with naming alcohol may tap into this old collection of perceptions and judgments.

How early do you start talking with children about their FASD?

As early as possible, in a way that's developmentally appropriate. Validating how they are as normal for themselves may help prevent frustration and increase understanding between parents and children. Talking about FASD optimally includes talking about strengths, and how all people have different challenges and strengths.

How do you talk with adolescents about their FASD?

First, think through the value of identification (i.e. to increase understanding, and to reduce confusion and frustration.) Identify your personal feelings about FASD, and if there is discomfort, find someone to talk with to help reduce discomfort since these feelings may complicate communication. Identify the person's strengths, and evaluate the person for the appropriateness of the timing of talking about FASD. Adolescents may reject any information that reinforces their fears that they are "less than" their peers, which suggests the importance of considering the context within which these discussions take place. If you are a concerned professional, involve parents in the process of talking. Remember also to ask if it is possible that the parents may have FASD themselves.

Don't children with FASD get angry with their parents when they find out about FASD?

Most people feel relief and grief. As one adolescent said, "Thank God. That means *I'm* not the problem, I *have* a problem. I can deal with that." When anger comes up, it may reflect the feelings of the adults who are introducing the information and how it is introduced, or it may involve feelings of loss. Anger is part of a grieving process and is addressable.

Aren't most adolescents with FASD violent and aggressive?

No, however, the longer there has been a poor fit, the greater the potential for chronic frustration. When frustration accumulates, emotional fuses seem shorter and shorter. The secondary characteristics of anger and aggression are not inevitable and are not always present in people with FASD.

Can people with FASD ever get married and have kids?

Yes, and some make wonderful parents. Others may continue to need support in order to be successful parents. Parenting may not be a good option for others, as is true for some people in the general population.

I hear people say that we have to "toughen the kids up" and prepare them for the "real world." We can't baby them, since after high school they have to fit in if they're going to succeed.

Children, adolescents and adults with FASD *are* in the real world. They just happen to have a handicapping condition that doesn't simply go away because they grow older. Just like people who need wheelchairs in the "real world," not just at home, people with FASD may need to continue to have appropriate supports. This suggests the importance of providing information about FASD to entire communities in order to assure continued support. There may be no facet of a community for whom this information is irrelevant; this includes parents, schools, medical, social and mental health services, employers and the judicial system.

GLOSSARY OF TERMS

Anomalies–Differences from the normal, especially as a result of congenital (dating from birth) or hereditary defects.

ARND–Alcohol-Related Neurodevelopmental Disorders: includes "Evidence of CNS neurodevelopmental abnormalities..." and/or "Evidence of a complex pattern of behavior or cognitive abnormalities that are inconsistent with developmental level and cannot be explained by familial background or environment alone, such as learning difficulties; deficits in school performance; poor impulse control; problems in social perception; deficits in higher level receptive and expressive language; poor capacity for abstraction or metacognition; specific deficits in mathematical skills, or problems in memory, attention, or judgment" (Institute of Medicine, 1996).

Atrial/Ventricular Defects– Defects in the heart's chambers. The upper two chambers of the heart are called the atria, the bottom two the ventricles.

CNS–Central Nervous System: the brain and spinal cord.

Camptodactyly–One or more fingers and/or toes remaining flexed or bent at one or more joints. Permanent bending of fingers or toes.

Clinodactyly–Abnormal bending of fingers or toes, permanent bending to the side, medially or laterally, of one or more fingers or toes.

Congenital–Existing at or dating from birth (i.e. congenital heart lesions are structural abnormalities of the heart that are present at birth, and develop during gestation).

Craniofacial–Having to do with the head and face region.

Dysmorphology–The study of birth defects or malformations.

Dysmorphologist–One who is knowledgeable about deviations from the normal physical patterns of development.

Embryo–Early stage of growth: the fertilized ovum, which eventually becomes the offspring during the period of most rapid development. In humans this period is from two weeks after fertilization until the end of the 7th or 8th week, after which time it is known as a fetus.

Epicanthal Folds–Vertical fold of skin on either side of the nose, covering the inner corner of the eye. Present as a normal characteristic associated with some races, it sometimes occurs as a congenital anomaly in others (i.e. FASD).

Epidemiology–Study of the incidence of a disease in a population and factors that influence it; goals of these studies are to find ways to prevent the disease.

Ethanol–The type of alcohol found in wine, beer and hard liquor.

Facies–Term used in anatomical language to designate: A) the face, and B) a specific surface of a body structure, part, or organ.

FAE–Fetal Alcohol Effects: various detrimental effects caused by exposure to alcohol during gestation in individuals who cannot be identified as having full fetal alcohol syndrome. This is the older term, predating both ARND and the new term, FASD.

FAS–Fetal Alcohol Syndrome: a specific, although variable, constellation of abnormalities that include facial features, growth retardation, and central nervous (brain) abnormalities.

FASD–Fetal Alcohol Spectrum Disorders refer to a range of birth defects that can include distinctive facial features, growth deficits, central nervous system involvement and a range of physical problems. This term was introduced in 2003 to encompass FAS, FAE, and ARND.

Fetus–Unborn offspring of an animal in the postembryonic period after major structures have been outlined; in humans, from the 7th or 8th week after fertilization until birth.

Gestation–The period of development in animals from the time of fertilization of the ovum until birth.

Heterotopias–Cells or tissue present in a place where it usually is not found. Heterotopias result from abnormalities of migration of cells during embryonic and fetal development.

Hirsutism–Abnormal hairiness.

Hypolasia–Incomplete development of an organ or structure resulting in small size.

IUGR–Intrauterine growth retardation: slower than average growth of a developing fetus. Such babies are born smaller than would be expected for their gestational age.

Malmigrations–Abnormal movement of cells or tissues during early embryonic development.

Maxillary Hypoplasia–Incomplete development of the bone of the upper jaw.

Metabolite–A substance which is produced through some chemical process in the body.

Micrognathia–Smaller than normal chin (see Relative Prognathia).

Microcephaly–Abnormally small circumference of the head.

Microopthalmia–Abnormal smallness of the eyes.

Motility–Ability to move spontaneously.

Neonate–Newborn under 28 days of age.

Organogenesis–The formation of organs (digestive tract, liver, heart, etc.) in the developing embryo. This occurs during the 3rd to 9th week of pregnancy in humans.

Palmar Creases–Any of the normal grooves across the palm which accommodate flexion of the hand.

Palpebral Fissure–Openings of the eyes; eye slits.

Parity–Number of live births delivered by a woman.

Pathogen—Specific causative agent of disease.

Perinatal—Period shortly before and after birth, generally considered to begin with completion of 28 weeks of gestation and ending 1 to 4 weeks after birth.

Philtrum—Vertical groove which runs from under the nose to the upper lip.

Placenta—Organ surrounding the fetus during pregnancy which joins the mother and fetus and supports growth and development during gestation.

Postnatal—After birth.

Prenatal—Before birth.

Prospective Study—A research study that designates beforehand a set of individuals who will be identified and followed over a course of time (see also: Retrospective Study).

Ptosis—Drooping of the upper eyelids.

Relative Prognathia—Lower jaw overgrows the upper jaw, often seen during adolescence where there is maxillary hypoplasia and the lower jaw grows at a genetically predetermined rate.

Retrospective Study—A research study that looks back at the past records of a designated set of individuals in an attempt to answer questions about health concerns.

Spermatogenesis—Producing semen or sperm.

Strabismus—Deviation or crossing of the eye; the inability of both eyes to focus on one object.

Syndrome—Group of characteristic features caused by one underlying process; the features present allow identification of individuals as having a unique and specific disorder.

Tachycardia—Rapid pulse; abnormal acceleration of heart beat.

Teratogen—Agent or factor which may cause abnormalities of development or differentiation in an embryo or fetus.

Teratogenesis–The disturbed processes that occur due to the exposure of a fetus to a teratogen.

Threshold Effect–No effects are seen below a certain level of exposure.

Toxemia–Metabolic disturbance in pregnancy characterized by hypertension (high blood pressure) and edema (swelling or fluid retention).

Toxin–Poisonous substance.

Tremulous–Shaking, trembling, or quivering.

Trimester–Three terms of three months each representing the nine months of pregnancy.

Vermillion–Bright red pigmentation or color. Lips are often referred to as the "vermillion border," which is often thinned in the upper lip of people with FASD.

RESOURCES

Advocacy

Knowledge and understanding are the basis for advocacy. For current research articles, search PubMed online or contact your local library or medical school library. Use search terms such as: Fetal Alcohol Syndrome, Fetal Alcohol Spectrum Disorders, Alcohol-Related Neurodevelopmental Disorders, Alcohol and Pregnancy Outcome, or search the specific names of other drugs.

About Diagnosis

There are few resources for diagnoses of FASD. Giving equal weight to the idea that brain function is the source of behaviors is important, and this increases understanding of the person even before there is a formal diagnosis. The most appropriate and informative diagnosis is done by a multi-disciplinary team. Optimally, this includes a neuropsychologist, a physician or nurse practitioner, an occupational therapist, and a social worker. Together, they are able to assess areas of functioning that may be affected by alcohol.

Services

FASCETS, Inc. – Parent, professional, agency and community information, consultation, education, support and program development. Our mission is *"To increase understanding of people from a neurobehavioral perspective."* FASCETS is a 501 (c)(3) nonprofit corporation. For information about our services, please contact: wtemko@fascets.org or call: 503-621-1271.

Websites

FASCETS, Inc. (Fetal Alcohol Syndrome Consultation, Education and Training Services, Inc.) www.fascets.org

NOFAS (National Organization on Fetal Alcohol Syndrome) www.nofas.org

SELECT BIBLIOGRAPHY

Behnke, M., & Smith, V. (2013) Technical report prenatal substance abuse: Short- and long-term effects on the exposed fetus. *American Academy of Pediatrics,* doi: www.pediatrics.org/cgi/doi/10.1542/peds.2012-3931

Clarren, S.K., & Astley, S.J. (2004) *Diagnostic Guide for Fetal Alcohol Spectrum Disorders: The 4–Digit Diagnostic Code.* University of Washington; Seattle, WA

Claire, D., Coles, K., Platzman, A., Raskind-Hood, L., Brown, R., Falek, A., & Smith, I. (1997) A comparison of children affected by prenatal alcohol exposure and attention deficit disorder. *Alcoholism: Clinical and Experimental Research,* 21(1), 150-161

Day, J., Soham, S., Savani, S., Krempley, B.D., Nguyen, M., & Kitlinska, J. (2016) Influence of paternal preconception exposures on their offspring: Through epigenetics to phenotype. *American Journal of Stem Cells 2016,* 5(1):11-18

Friedler, G. (1988) Effects on future generations of paternal exposure to alcohol and other drugs. *Alcohol Health and Research World,* 12(2), 126–129

Kleinfeld, J. & Wescott, S. (1993) *Fantastic Antone Succeeds: Experiences in Educating Children with Fetal Alcohol Syndrome.* University of Alaska Press, Fairbanks, AK

Malbin, D., Boulding, D., & Brooks, S. (2010) Trying differently: Rethinking juvenile justice using a neuro-behavioral model. *American Bar Association Juvenile Justice Committee Newsletter,* (5)

Malbin, D. (2015) *Fetal Alcohol / Neurobehavioral Conditions: Understanding and Application of a Brain-Based Approach – A Collection of Information for Parents and Professionals, Third Edition.* Available through FASCETS, Inc., www.fascets.org

McBride, N., & Johnson, S. (2016) Fathers' role in alcohol-exposed pregnancies. *Systematic Review of Human Studies,* 51(2), 240–248

Petrenko, C., Pandolfino, M., & Roddenbery, R. (2016) The association between parental attributions of misbehavior and parenting practices in caregivers raising children with prenatal alcohol exposure: A mixed-methods study. *Research in Developmental Disabilities,* 59, 255-267

Shaywitz, S.E., Cohen, D.J., & Shaywitz, B.A. (1980) Behavior and learning difficulties in children of normal intelligence born to alcoholic mothers. *The Journal of Pediatrics,* 95(6) 978–982

Streissguth, A.P., & Kanter, J. (1996) Primary and secondary disabilities in fetal alcohol syndrome. *The Challenge of Fetal Alcohol Syndrome: Overcoming Secondary Disabilities:* University of Washington Press, Seattle, WA

Yazigi, R.A., Odem, R.R., & Polakoski, K.L. (1991) Demonstration of specific binding of Cocaine to human spermatozoa. *Journal of the American Medical Association,* 266 (14), 1956-1959

APPENDIX

Diagnostic Criteria for Fetal Alcohol Syndrome (FAS) and Alcohol-Related Effects

Fetal Alcohol Syndrome

1. FAS with confirmed maternal alcohol exposure
   A. Confirmed maternal alcohol exposure
   B. Evidence of a characteristic pattern of facial anomalies that includes features such as short palpebral fissures and abnormalities in the premaxillary zone (e.g. flat upper lip, flattened philtrum, and flat midface.)
   C. Evidence of growth retardation, as in at least one of the following:
      • Low birth weight for gestational age
      • Decelerating weight over time not due to nutrition
      • Disproportional low weight to height
   D. Evidence of CNS neurodevelopmental abnormalities, as in at least one of the following:
      • Decreased cranial size at birth
      • Structural brain abnormalities (e.g. microcephaly, partial or complete agenesis of the corpus callosum, cerebellar hypoplasia)
      • Neurological hard or soft signs (as age proportionate), such as impaired fine motor skills, neurosensory hearing loss, poor tandem gait, poor eye-hand coordination
2. FAS without confirmed maternal alcohol exposure
   B, C, and D as above

3. Partial FAS with confirmed maternal alcohol exposure
   A. Confirmed maternal alcohol exposure
   B. Evidence of some components of the pattern of characteristic facial anomalies either C or D or E
   C. Evidence of growth retardation, as in at least one of the following:
      • low birth weight for gestational age
      • decelerating weight over time not due to nutrition
      • disproportionate low weight to height
   D. Evidence of CNS neurodevelopmental abnormalities, as in:
      • decreased cranial size at birth
      • structural brain abnormalities (e.g. microcephaly, partial or complete agenesis of the corpus callosum, cerebellar hypoplasia)
      • neurological hard or soft signs (as age appropriate) such as impaired fine motor skills, neurosensory hearing loss, poor tandem gait, poor eye-hand coordination
   E. Evidence of a complex pattern of behavior or cognitive abnormalities that are inconsistent with developmental level and cannot be explained by familial background or environment alone, such as learning difficulties; deficits in school performance; poor impulse control; problems in social perception; deficits in higher level receptive and expressive language; poor capacity for abstraction or metacognition; specific deficits in mathematical skills; or problems in memory, attention, or judgement

Alcohol-Related Effects

Clinical conditions in which there is a history of maternal alcohol exposure, and where clinical or animal research has linked maternal alcohol ingestion to an observed outcome. There are two categories, which may co-occur. If both diagnoses are present, then both diagnoses should be rendered:

Alcohol-related birth defects (ARBD)

4. List of congenital anomalies, including malformations and dysplasias

Cardiac	Atrial septal defects Ventricular septal defects	Aberrant great vessels Teratology of Fallot
Skeletal	Hypoplastic nails Shortened fifth digits Radioulnar synostosis Flexion contractures Camptodactyly	Clinodactyly Pectus excavatum and carinatum Klippel-Feil syndrome Hemivertebrae Scoliosis
Renal	Aplastic, dysplastic Hypoplastic kidneys Horseshoe kidneys	Ureteral duplications Hydronephrosis
Ocular	Strabismus	Refractive problems secondary to small globes Retinal vascular anomalies
Auditory	Conductive hearing loss	Neurosensory hearing loss
Other	Virtually every malformation has been described in some patient with FAS. The etiological specificity of most of these anomalies to alcohol teratogensesis remains uncertain.	

5. Alcohol-related neurodevelopmental disorder (ARND)

Presence of:

A. Evidence of CNS neurodevelopmental abnormalities, as in any one of the following:
  • decreased cranial size at birth
  • structural brain abnormalities (e.g., microcephaly, partial or complete agenesis of the corpus callosum, cerebellar hypoplasia)
  • neurological hard or soft signs (as age appropriate), such as impaired fine motor skills, neurosensory hearing loss, poor tandem gait, poor eye-hand coordination

and/or:

B. Evidence of a complex pattern of behavior or cognitive abnormalities that are inconsistent with developmental level and cannot be explained by familial background or environment alone, such as learning difficulties; deficits in school performance; poor impulse control; problems in social perception; deficits in higher level receptive and expressive language; poor capacity for abstraction or metacognition; specific deficits in mathematical skills; or problems in memory, attention, or judgement

Source: Stratton, K., Howe, C., and Battaglia, F., (Editors): Fetal Alcohol Syndrome; Diagnosis Epidemiology, Prevention, and Treatment; National Academy Press, Washington, DC, 1996